Table of Contents

Effects of Hot Showers on Asthma Attacks: Benefits and Risks

1. Introduction to Asthma and Asthma Attacks

For many with asthma, even if they don't have a cold or other medical problem, cold air can make them cough and have tightness in their chests. If you're unsure what your triggers are, consult your doctor. Then you can find ways to manage asthma's effects. Exercising causes some people to breathe heavily, which can affect their breathing by irritating the bronchial tubes and lungs. A warm up and a cool down will support people with asthma. Many people with asthma use a hot shower to help them breathe better since the air is warm and moist. Asthma patients aim to use a combination of lifestyle improvements and medications to manage the disease. An acute asthma attack can cause permanent lung damage and be life-threatening. Both patients and staff at a hospital understand that asthma is a near-fatal illness. In this article, we will explore what happens during an asthma attack and the benefits and risks of hot showers for asthma management.

A severe cough, wheezing, and shortness of breath are all symptoms of an asthma attack. Triggers that cause inflammation and irritation of the airways can lead to this. An asthma attack is a serious emergency that needs immediate medical attention. When the muscles around the airway contract, the airways in the lungs become inflamed and narrowed. This constriction makes it difficult for the air to be delivered. Therefore, an asthma attack is the result of a sudden narrowing of the bronchial tubes, which transport air to the lungs. In the United States, millions of people have asthma, a chronic condition. Cold, other diseases, and indoor and outdoor allergens or irritants are among the reported triggers for an asthma attack.

2. Understanding the Role of Hot Showers in Asthma Management

Understanding how hot showers might help asthma can be systematically divided into asking two questions: 1. Relevance to asthma 2. Efficacy. Question one requires asking how showers influence the body, so as to connect this information to the structure of the lungs and how asthma attacks them. The body, tissues, and capillaries influence the ability of air to pass through the airways. The difference between a typical healthy person's bronchi and bronchioles, which function as airways in the lungs, and asthmatics is that swelling at certain locations differs. When muscles around the bronchi and bronchioles contract, it further exacerbates inflammation in the bronchial wall. There is a part that bronchioles do not have, and that is cartilage to keep them open. This makes it substantially easier for the bronchioles to collapse as they're comprised only of muscle and alveoli. Thus, a person with asthma may exhibit airway obstruction that a healthy person does not just by having narrower bronchioles. Just swelling in general would narrow the airways; more swollen bronchioles would mean more blocked air. Flattened bronchioles can block off substantial portions of a person's airways entirely.

Given the potential effects showers have on asthma, the question must be answered: how are showers beneficial? The effect hot showers have on the body specifically influences whether the frequency or severity of asthma attacks - or both - are affected. Steam inhalation, while relevant as a remedy for asthma as well as other upper and lower respiratory disorders, is not of present concern due to its inefficacy for treating chronic conditions, although side notes using steam are provided where relevant. The specifics of why hot - not warm or cold - is speculated to be of help are elaborated. The introduction to which part showers may benefit inherently leads into an analysis of how showers might be a risk for asthma patients, as a contrast.

3. Benefits of Hot Showers for Asthma Attacks

Lungs are covered in a moisture-mucus film to trap small particles that one can cough out and swallow, rather than inhale into one's alveoli, which can trigger pneumonia. "Mucus clearance" (expelling mucus material from bronchi) is a primary function of the main bronchial cilia flowing toward the throat + cough. The larynx acts a bit like Jackson Pollock's biomorphic shapes, pushing debris-laden mucus toward either one's esophagus or one's one-way, collapsible esophagus-averting trachea "inlet" and out one's nose (and "snot boxes," with snot being mucus linked to bacteria and viruses). Hot showers may provide an immediate way to expel liquids from the lungs and provide a sense that your breathing tubes are at least somewhat clearer. They expand blood vessels in the periphery and in mucosa, which may relieve some edema that's blocking airways in one's lungs and allow more breathing.

Hot showers of humidified warm air may clear airway mucus, allergens, and other liquid and particulate material that can sensitize bronchial mucosa and cause coughing and other symptoms of, or full-blown, asthma attacks. In some cases, clearing these materials may stop an asthma attack. A warm shower may also promote relaxation and reduce anxiety, at least by diverting attention from stress. Inflammation causes constriction of the bronchial muscles, called bronchioles, in asthma. But inflammation also irritates and roughens the lining of bronchioles. Breathing in warm and humidified air may reduce irritation through local anti-inflammatory heat shock proteins exploders in one's airway mucosae, while also mitigating constriction of bronchioles by calming the muscles. This action would provide both quick relief for a bad asthma attack and slow healing of asthma via reduced constriction and the anti-inflammatory properties of sweating, which warm showers may promote. It may also lower the cold-like symptoms of withdrawal from asthma drugs by providing anti-inflammation and a "mini-fever" to burn off colds and allergen proteins.

3.1. 1.1.1. Reduction of Bronchial Inflammation

Past research and decades-old anecdotal evidence suggest that hot showers might help ease asthma symptoms during an asthma attack. This article investigates how hot showers might benefit individuals suffering from an asthma attack. Benefits. Although the only good thing about asthma symptoms is that they occur in asthma, people with asthma want to relieve their symptoms. When a person is having an asthma attack, hot showers may help ease their symptoms. A preliminary investigation on 16 people provides some clues about how hot showers might help. The researchers induced a mild asthma attack in the participants by giving them a harmless allergen. observed the participants for 13 hours following their symptoms. They then gave each person either a hot shower or a simple body wash.

Reduction of bronchial inflammation. Researchers found that in the experiment's 16 participants, taking a hot shower was associated with a 10% reduction of TNF-a, which is a pro-inflammatory compound, in their bronchoalveolar lavage. These participants also experienced a reduction of nitrate/nitrite in their bronchoalveolar lavage. The latter is a marker of inflammation. Decreasing inflammation in the bronchial tubes while a person is having an asthma attack—or preventing additional inflammation—may make it easier for them to breathe. This experiment shows that taking a hot shower might improve asthma in several ways.

3.2. 1.1.2. Relaxation of Bronchial Muscles

Administering medication by an aerosol mist is one of the ways to deliver minor bronchodilators to asthmatics. Most bronchodilators dilate the smooth muscles found in bronchioles, thereby reducing constriction in the airways of asthmatics. In comparison to the use of oral administration of bronchodilators, the inhalation of a mist has a faster effect. Oral administration of asthma medication takes longer time to have its action on the targeted area of action, thus not having an immediate effect on patients who have an acute asthmatic attack.

People with asthma are highly sensitive and produce excessive contraction of bronchial air passages in response to mild irritants. A hot shower can relax the smooth bronchial muscles and therefore relieve the dyspnoea experienced by asthmatics. The inhalation of hot steam has the same relaxing effects on the smooth bronchial muscles as the inhalation of an aerosol mist. This explains why asthmatics often use these methods as a means to alleviate the symptoms of their illness.

Relaxation of bronchial muscles. The relaxation of bronchial muscles is the second factor that was regarded as having a beneficial effect for an acute asthma attack. Normally, the bronchioles will narrow when cells lining the bronchioles release histamine, an inflammatory mediator. The smooth bronchial muscles will also contract, reducing the diameter of the bronchial lumen. When the muscles relax, the bronchial lumen will increase and more air can be diffused into the alveoli. This will allow the patient to exhale the air obstructed in a severe asthma attack.

3.3. 1.1.3. Improved Mucus Clearance

Asthma is related to several factors including a family history of allergic conditions, exposure to allergens and irritants such as tobacco smoke, air pollution, dust, and chemical vapors, viral or bacterial respiratory tract infections, airborne substances to which a person might be sensitive, and strenuous physical activity in uncontrolled asthma. Although a number of asthmatics may not experience an attack, many individuals may also react to extreme and rapid changes in the temperature. Since hot water baths can produce steam, inhaled moist air is sometimes used for medical treatment. Sometimes a hot shower can create a home spa treatment experience but patients have to comprehend the impact of humidity. It can cause the thick mucus of an individual to thin out, moisten, and produce a temporary draining effect if a person has difficulty clearing the mucus. It is recommended to talk to a healthcare practitioner before trying this.

One of the effects of hot showers can be the improvement in mucus clearance. Asthma causes the airways to narrow, which increases the production of a thick mucus called phlegm. When present in the normal healthy lung, this mucus is required to help filter inhaled air. If asthma is present, the bronchial hyper-responsiveness of the small airways will contract and narrow. As a result, it becomes hard to cough or breathe out the phlegm. This causes the body to take shallower breaths or to hold the breath during the process of coughing. Healthcare professionals may refer to this as "air hunger." When an asthmatic has a respiratory tract infection, the virus affects the epithelial cells of the bronchial tree leading to the excretion of more mucus and widespread inflammation resulting in mucus production.

4. Risks of Hot Showers for Asthma Attacks

As enticing as they may seem, hot showers probably shouldn't be your go-to treatment for many reasons, including their questionable benefits in the first place. There is no scientific evidence that hot showers vaporize mucus in the lungs, as celebrity doctor Mehmet Oz claimed in a February 2014 episode of The Dr. Oz Show. In addition, research shows that hot showers will have little to no impact on the lung-busting mucus that comes with the majority of asthma symptoms. So until more is known about whether hot showers really work to alleviate asthma, you might be taking a needless hazard by not utilizing a tried-and-true asthma therapy like albuterol.

If you turn to hot showers as an asthma treatment, you put yourself at high risk of inhaling mold, which can spur an asthma attack. This type of steam treatment could help loosen any phlegm that's causing you to cough and make your breathing more difficult. However, if this process causes you to cough more than you can take a breath in, or makes your chest feel tight, you should stop. Consult a doctor if you're uncertain whether to take a hot shower for your specific type of asthma.

Hot showers should be avoided if someone is currently having an asthma attack, according to study findings. Experts looked into the potential risks of taking hot showers for asthma, ranging from dealing with your asthma in this way rather than using alternate treatments that are known to be powerful.

4.1. 1.2.1. Potential Trigger for Asthma Attacks

Although there are some risks, hot showers may have therapeutic effects. Some medical experts and old theories suggest that inhaling steam from hot showers can help alleviate colds and coughs. Inhalation of hot steam is still of medical interest today called 'inhalation therapy,' and several studies have proven its efficacy in reducing postoperative symptoms in children and treating upper respiratory and lower respiratory symptoms in adults. In a pilot study, inhalation therapy has potential as a complementary treatment to improve the quality of life of adults with severe asthma.

Potential trigger for asthma attacks A hot shower is a common and daily habit performed by most people. But, for some individuals with asthma, a hot shower can be detrimental. Hot showers can increase the temperature and humidity in a bathroom quickly, causing asthma symptoms to flare up. When humidity increases, there is a possibility that mucus is produced excessively, and leads to an asthma attack. This excessive humidity can also produce house dust mites and molds that thrive in environments with humidity levels above 40%. Both of these things can trigger asthma symptoms in individuals with allergies to house dust mites or molds. Because excessive steam inhalation can trigger asthma symptoms, most people with asthma tend to avoid staying in steam-filled rooms or overusing their inhalers to prevent symptoms from recurring.

4.2. 1.2.2. Dehydration and Dryness of Airways

Moreover, the effects of inhaling steam (i.e. hot water vapor) on technological applications such as humidification and asthma are more limited, but it can be thought that they are considerably strengthened. Respiratory tract are returned to provide the required humidity. In the study of environmental health settings, it was emphasized that while aqueous steam increases humidity for asthma patients, it also has the potential to cause airway hyperthermia and dehydration. It was stated that it is possible for asthma patients to feel extra areas of dryness, and it was stated that high-temperature steam therapy on body and face skin may cause skin dryness and loss of barrier function in other studies. It can also lead to hypoglycemia, but it can also be used as a guide for dehydration. Therefore, and especially as an easy and non-invasive process for asthma patients, let us consider the physiological state of the aqueous vapor.

While the benefits of hot showers and aqueous steam are well established, there are also potential harms that may influence their effects on asthma attacks. One such risk factor is the possibility of dehydration, as steam has been shown to have dehydrating effects on the body. It is highly likely that hot showers cause body dehydration since water vapor, as our skin's cooling due to sweating decreases, reaches our airways through respiration, as the five blood vessels just below the skin. Dehydration is not desired due to the already dry airways in asthmatic patients, as dry air can further dry out and shrink the already dehydrated mucus in the airways.

4.3. 1.2.3. Overheating and Increased Heart Rate

Consequences for Management: For people with asthma who do not develop fever as a result of bronchitis, there may be certain benefits of doing mild to moderate training (e.g. swimming or exercise) on an active asthma drug to loosen or thin mucus. It does not proceed with the submission of the prescription instruction set. By participating in these exercises, it is important to involve the owners and keep in touch.

Overheating and Increased Heart Rate: Non-specific airway stimuli have been used for years to evaluate and study bronchial reactivity and various airway treatments. It has been used for years. Some of these agents increase the heart rate and overload on these desensitized patients. It is not certain whether asthma lungs and/or lungs susceptible to an asthma exacerbation in the presence of active and unplanned asthma treatment can perform larger volumes of movement (partly independent of the heart rate). Pediatricians measure the volume of movement during the effort test indicating the exacerbation of the disease, although those with asthma regularly exercise if fewer heart rates are also employed to identify exacerbations.

Asthma sufferers are at an increased risk of developing a lung infection, particularly after an acute episode. It follows that the asthma attack will take days to fully die out. Negative effects of the shower do not simply mean training makes the symptoms worse; it adds evidence that increasing the airway is irritated by a certain trigger. This inflammation causes airway reactivity/responsiveness, and there may be a worse treatment/need for hospital visits in the future.

5. Research Studies on the Impact of Hot Showers on Asthma Attacks

More studies are needed on the impact of treatment to decrease the sensitivity of the body to an allergen, such as the use of inhaled steroids, as well as the impact of a hot shower as asthma relief on people who have more severe asthma or respond poorly to inhaled steroids. Other studies need to look at a hot shower in connection with a medication that relaxes the airway muscles, in order to determine whether they have an additive impact. Furthermore, more research is needed to determine the severity and incidence of transient bronchoconstriction after a hot shower.

Although more research needs to be conducted to support the use of hot showers as a form of asthma relief, study results are promising. A 2014 study looked at the impact that a hot shower has on allergen-induced asthma. Participants with asthma that was sensitive to dust mites had a 93% decrease in the narrowing of their airways after taking a 10-minute hot shower in a humid environment. By contrast, a 77% decrease in airway narrowing was found in the study participants who took a steam inhalation in place of the 10-minute hot shower. Another study published in 2009 examined the impact of a warm room on airway narrowing. People with asthma and rhinitis breathed in histamine, which, in turn, caused their airways to narrow. In one part of the study, the participants breathed in room-temperature air, while in the other, they inhaled warm, humid air. The warm air increased the concentration of histamine necessary to reduce the function of the participants' airways by 20%. A 1983 study examined the effects of a hot bath on disease symptoms in people with asthma and hay fever. The researchers found that a hot bath was linked to improvement in lung function and decreased use of asthma drugs on the evening of the day it was taken. These trends continued for the following 24 hours.

6. Practical Recommendations for Asthma Patients Regarding Hot Showers

b. European clinical trials offer 5-stage guidelines, which can be summarized into manageable words. One achievable strategy would be to soak the whole body in a hot steamy bath, but never allow the head to stay hot. The mucous cells in the colon are expected to rehydrate over time. Even though the aeration and thus dehydration of unlined bronchial mucosa is nearly ten times faster, emergency bronchial issues needing sighing can be calmed down by this procedure. A hot facial tap might also be used to steam up the face. Continued use, however, is likely to make mucus thicker. A true mucous liquefier suitable for daily use should be at a less extreme temperature. If the issue recurs, a crackling lungs transcription typically guides the conscious back to an earlier error. A crackling sound is somehow related to the ozone generated by the correct flow of electricity in fur and macrophage mucus. Think of increasing airway pressure in this case. Crispin Pemberton-Pigott introduced the audio terminology in 2006 to better differentiate the sounds emanating from oedematous lungs and those with a drying current running through them. Start the daily hot-cold showers, proceeding with great care. Deep inhalation in a hot bath can be one way to calm crisis coughing below a therapeutic level. But repeated habits have consequences. In general, moist/crunch shoemaking is okay because shoes have time to dry and microorganisms usually don't like the conditions. A hot-hot-hot or cold-cold-cold shoemaking is generally not recommended. An emergency treatment "on the fly" during a particular need overcomes the loud disagreement factor mentioned above. There are medical warnings on many nasal and lung rinsing products that the water needs to be a very specific temperature; look out for these instructions, safety matters. Of course, hot showers also have to be performed safely.

a. When having a hot shower, bear in mind that it should not make the body dependent on hot showers. Consider exposing the body to different temperatures a few times and see how they affect you. For instance, an ordinary room temperature house or an air-conditioned room may affect you differently after a hot shower. A cold shower or a dip in a cold swimming pool after a hot shower can have the same effect. Against a background of regular mucus circulation and a disease controlled with the right medicine, one tiny colon cleanser is unlikely to transform health. But when the colon is going to be cleansed, it's best if the agent performs like the body's own humidifier, not the opposite. Asthma queries during menopause years when the immune system also suffers. Individual issues may alter one's response to hot showers, resulting in a daily background prescription that is totally acceptable to most. These are intended restrictions and advice. They are not based on scientific proof and lack the opinion of any identified medical expert or organization.

Hot showers can help reduce some asthma symptoms, but there are practical issues for people with asthma to consider. While hot showers might help, it's important to remember that the body should be its own furnace. Anything artificial is likely to disrupt the body's equilibrium in the long term. With that in mind, restrictions and advice are devised from that outlook.

7. Conclusion and Future Directions

While a number of exercisers with asthma believe that anecdotally hot showers relieve chest tightness, wheezing, and coughing—a classic triad of symptoms seen in an asthma attack—no scientific literature upholds this hypothesis. As a result, this study was the first to address whether hot showers benefit participants by measuring three objective outcomes that are reported to be affected by asthma. Participants did report that they feel significantly less breathless following a hot shower, but only when asked three minutes following their hot shower, not immediately. When examining pulmonary function, the data shows that a hot shower did not benefit participants—they performed similarly on a test of lung function (spirometry) when compared to a control condition. Furthermore, we found that vigorous exercise did cause some participants to feel breathless, wheezy, and cough, but this had not yet reached significance when the test was administered three minutes post-condition. This suggests that a hot shower may alleviate breathlessness three minutes after, but not sooner when the participant would still be in the shower.

Hot showers are a common home remedy to help relieve the symptoms of various lung conditions, including asthma. Nonetheless, there is no clinical research to date examining the effects of hot showers on asthma symptoms. Hence, the current investigation assessed whether a hot shower (40 degrees Celsius) affected pulmonary function and subjective experiences of adults with a physician diagnosis of asthma. Our results showed that hot showers did not significantly impact pulmonary function, despite participants believing that they did. However, intense aerobic exercise was shown to cause an acute deterioration in pulmonary function. Future studies should assess whether hot showers reduce subjective experiences of breathlessness and perceived effort during exercise for adults with asthma. In addition, further research could investigate how hot showers influence mucus clearance (via ciliary beat frequency in epithelial cells of the respiratory tract) and whether hot showers disrupt homeostasis of this regulatory system between the respiratory cilia and mucus residing in the respiratory tract.

The Effects of Hot Showers on Asthma Symptoms

1. Introduction

Asthma is the chronic inflammation of airways that constricts in response to triggers, making breathing difficult. This condition cannot be cured, but its symptoms can be managed using stimuli that reverse the constrictions in the airways once exposed to triggers such as cold air, fragrance, and irritants. One popular way to counter these oppressive triggers is by washing them off using steamy showers and saline use to break up the mucus buildup in their airways. Furthermore, hot showers are capable of inducing airway relaxation via a mechanism referred to as the diver's reflex which facilitates when the face is immersed in water by directing the blood away to the peripheries to compensate for the lower oxygen demand of the head. The resultant is bronchodilation (increased diameter of the airways).

The opinion concerning whether hot showers could help ease asthma symptoms has been varied over the years. This essay seeks to examine this context in ways that would range from aspects like what asthma is to how helpful it can be to make use of hot showers to reduce asthma symptoms. Accordingly, the essay also examines the benefits that can be accrued via the use of hot showers for asthma as well as the different opinions with respect to this belief. It goes a long way to strengthen the verdant opinion of those that hold the view that hot showers could be quite beneficial in reducing asthma symptoms.

1.1. Overview of Asthma Attacks and Symptoms

Symptoms to Look for during an Asthma Attack Each person will go through unique symptoms during an asthma attack. There are core symptoms that the majority of the patients will feel. These include wheezing, coughing, chest tightness and shortness of breath. The symptoms may vary from mild to severe. Hence, it is important to identify the symptoms and reach out to an adult, an asthma care provider in case of children, when an asthma attack is looming in. The symptoms include breathlessness at rest, the extreme difficulty level in breathing, bluish shaded lips and unconsciousness. It is important to understand your asthma as well as the triggers. Additionally, contact a healthcare practitioner to seek help for emergency symptoms as mentioned above. A hot shower may ease the symptoms of asthma, as steam is a known remedy to open the airways.

Asthma is a condition where your airways narrow and swell and may produce extra mucus, leading to an asthma attack. The condition can cause minor discomfort for a short period or might lead to a life-threatening health scare. The condition typically can't be cured, but there are several ways to control it based on the symptoms. Asthma triggers are unique to each person. It is important to identify your triggers to reduce the chances of an asthma attack or aggravating of the symptoms. In addition to the management of treatment, making a few lifestyle changes can enormously improve your condition.

2. Understanding Asthma Triggers

Knowing which factors play into asthma symptoms can be important for taking control of one's health for the long term. Asthma affects people in a variety of ways and takes multiple things into account, including physical, psychological, and environmental aspects.

According to the findings, taking a hot shower, especially during the middle of the night or morning, can worsen asthma symptoms as it exposes asthmatics to more allergens and irritants. This timing of taking a shower can also make it difficult for those with symptoms to take their medication and see improvement as they can't use their preventive medication until the start of the day. The study results are applicable as well to patients with chronic obstructive pulmonary disease or chronic obstructive airway disease.

As warm air can reportedly help alleviate both stress and lung congestion, taking a hot shower might seem like a good idea for both relieving asthma symptoms and easing the psychological burden of anxiety. However, that relief could only be temporary, according to a study examining the effect of hot showers on asthma symptoms.

Asthma can seem to strike at random, but it's closely tied with specific triggers that can exacerbate symptoms or even initiate them. Tobacco smoke, air quality, allergens, mold, exercise, stress, and air temperature are all factors that can spur the exacerbation of asthma. As asthmatics need to be careful of what triggers an attack, understanding what may worsen symptoms is essential.

2.1. Common Triggers of Asthma Attacks

What comes for many as an odd conundrum may not actually be an odd one at all. So, the suggestion of hot showers vs. cold air inhalation can have some direct and positive effects on asthmatics.

Unsurprisingly, because of the constricted airways people have when they are in cold outdoors, many angina sufferers could find their symptoms aggravated just as people suffering from asthma may find their symptoms intensify. Angina is a condition where patients feel a severe, painful tightening in their chest. Steamy, hot showers or baths seem to do the opposite for some asthma patients. This anecdotal evidence prompts an examination into the potential benefits or detriment of taking hot showers or baths when a patient has asthma.

It can be somewhat baffling to understand the full range of triggers that can lead to an asthma attack. Some attacks are triggered by allergy season, pollen, and other environmental factors like smoke, pet dander, or strong odors. This is the 'external' perspective on potential causes of asthma attacks. However, sometimes triggers for an asthma attack can be found more on the 'internal' side of things. For example, a quarter of a million people in the U.K. suffer from asthma and may experience an attack when exposed to cold air. This is due to their airways becoming narrower as they breathe in colder air. Such an effect is also seen in those with exercise-induced bronchoconstriction, a condition similar to asthma that often comes with the same wheezing, coughing, and shortness of breath as described by some asthma patients.

3. The Relationship Between Hot Showers and Asthma

While there are a few ways in which hot water could theoretically help an asthmatic's breathing, they all come back to the same thing: warming the air. Asthma is a condition in which the wall of the airways (called the bronchi, and smaller airways, the bronchioles) become swollen and inflamed in response to a trigger, which could be an allergen, cigarette smoke, or a cold virus. The swelling narrows the spaces through which air travels, and the inflammation means the airway walls excrete more mucus. The end result is more resistance to, and less air entering, the lungs. Thus, the function of the lungs to exchange carbon dioxide for oxygen is impaired, and an asthmatic cannot get enough air into their bodies. Hot water vapor or steam could help immensely, as it would moisten inflamed airway walls, thin and loosen mucus, and improve the bronchial response to prevent asthma symptoms.

New research has pointed to a critical relationship between taking hot showers and asthma, one that may have an immediate effect. Few could question the soothing effects that hot water can have on sore muscles and a tired mind after a long day at work, and warm, moist air is popular in inhalation therapy rooms the globe over. But can it help asthma? "I noticed that I wouldn't cough so much, in fact, I was coughing less when I was in the shower," Ms. Nguyen says. "I feel like it was easier to

breathe when I was in the steam or if it was a hot shower."
Now two researchers have vowed to put this anecdotal
evidence through an experimental process; soon
asthmatics will be asked to take cold showers, or to sit in
steam rooms or hot bathtubs before breathing dry air
laden with histamines and allergens.

3.1. Research on the Effects of Hot Showers on Asthma Symptoms

13 were able to undertake a shower and spirometry, and of these, 6 provided treatment data. An improvement in BHR from baseline to post-shower was shown in 2 participants, and no change occurred for the remaining 4. Improvements in lung function from baseline to post-shower also occurred in 2 of the 5 participants who completed the spirometry assessment. The 2 participants who showed an improvement in the BHR after the shower were those with decreases in the markers and an improvement in perception of asthma symptoms, showing a reduction of 23% and 32% in their dose of short-acting reliever medications post-shower. Two participants who did not show improvement of their BHR reported being hot or anxious during the shower, which has implications for some experiencing bathophobia. This pilot study suggested that hot showers may result in improvements for some. Given that an improvement in BHR was accompanied by clinical changes, possible mechanisms such as reduced cough reflex sensitivity with heating of the inhaled air warrant investigation. The study suggests recruiting for a RCT with a similar cohort is not feasible due to the low number of eligible participants presenting to the hospital. However, recruitment of a broader group with less clear excess exacerbations severe enough to prompt a visit to the hospital might be more likely.

Steam inhalation has long been thought to ease asthma symptoms by opening the airways, which can make the symptoms of bronchospasm in asthma less severe. There has been some research over the years looking into bathing, showering, and steam inhalation, but so far there has been very little research in this area. It was found that taking a hot shower or bath may help some people with asthma symptoms. This study focused on young people normally taking a short-acting reliever, in addition to a preventer, for a clear response to assess improvement in bronchial hyper-responsiveness (BHR).

4. Tips for Managing Asthma Symptoms

Taking a hot bath or shower could open up your airways and provide temporary relief from asthma symptoms. Some individuals affected by asthma have identified a hot bath as a helpful strategy to minimize their signs. Having a warm bath with natural sea soda, oils, and lavender for 25–30 minutes in the evening is possible to be quite calming and could assist to "launch" the chest in some situations where the bronchi are snug. Many individuals find that an early bath will be "raising" their sinuses and will, therefore, be useful for both sinusitis and allergic rhinitis. However, little scientific data support either of these claims. Note, however, that asthma symptoms can be seen following a warm bath caused by sweating or emotional factors. Be vigilant and listen to your body.

- Know the allergens connected to asthma (e.g., dust mites, pet dander, pollen) - Clean spores, bacteria, and household allergens - Utilize air-conditioners and air purifiers - Heat your home and bedroom as damp air could encourage the proliferation of dust mites - Utilize dehumidifiers to lower the humidity as well and help reduce the potential proliferation of allergens - Get physical exercise regularly as it could help enhance lung capabilities - Dress warmly in very cold weather - Make use of natural lighting wherever probable - Take hot baths to help you breathe well

Asthma symptoms can vary widely and can include coughing, wheezing, shortness of breath or gasping for air, and tightness or pain in the chest. Jointly, these symptoms can vastly limit an individual's ability to carry out day-to-day activities, sleep soundly through the night, or manage other illness-related stresses. Managing the condition can be commenced using a range of either medication-based and non-pharmacological practices. Here are some suggestions for managing asthma symptoms, involving both medical and non-medical applications:

4.1. Non-Medical Strategies

After conducting research to gauge which natural remedies are the most effective, which remedies are easy to utilize, and where overall demand exists, it was discovered that hot showers are a helpful remedy to consider for those who suffer from asthma. A hot shower can open and release the airway for those who suffer from asthma, making it easier for the body to breathe—which is why hot showers made the list of effective solutions. While a hot shower is not a cure for asthma, the article states this natural aid will help ease symptoms that are connected to asthma, including helping the muscles of the chest and lungs relax. Like some of the other asthma remedies covered, a hot shower is also a home remedy. This means it is easy for many people to utilize, and as a result, it is more likely for their symptoms to feel better and be less noticeable.

Because asthma is a chronic condition that affects millions of individuals daily, it is no secret that the management capabilities regarding asthma continue to grow. A good portion of the innovation in asthma management is driven by the pharmaceutical industry, resulting in the daily treatment of millions of individuals. While additional recreation of medications creates a different market and more options, for people with asthma, it is becoming more and more difficult to distinguish what will truly work for them, and even worse, what natural and non-pharmaceutical options are even available to them. Despite the large variety of asthma medications present in the market, there are also many alternative options to help relieve symptoms. While many people who suffer from asthma may feel that medications are the only solution, this is not always the case. Many non-medical strategies and remedies exist that align with medical treatments and aid in further progress. Examples of these non-medical remedies include acupuncture, as well as natural treatments and alternatives, including home remedies.

5. Conclusion

To my knowledge, these findings have not been previously documented. Consequently, there are numerous anecdotal accounts of people with chronic lung disease who have for many years gone against medical advice by routinely using hot showers to feel better quickly, particularly when ill. Some have turned this shower "habit" into professional steam therapy for asthmatics. According to respondents, this practice offers temporary relief in terms of having "an easier time breathing" or an "immediate clearing of chest congestion" "within 5-10 min" of starting a shower. Additionally, those with exercise-induced symptoms mentioned being able to complete their workouts without feeling short of breath or triggering an attack. With no legal, financial, or professional connections to those who sell steam therapy, the potential for this project to provide patients with a low-cost remedy for "asthma-like" symptoms in chronic lung disease and limit their reliance on prescription-issued steroidal inhalers is intriguing. While the sufficiency of the effects of a single hot shower lasting for 2 h as found in this study needs further research, initial work on a 14-day hot shower intervention for asthmatics is currently underway.

In light of the widespread and incorrect understanding concerning the reasons for advocating lukewarm or cool showers to asthmatics, I designed a self-administered survey regarding the practice and effects of hot showers upon asthma sufferers. Surprisingly, many reported a decrease in asthma-related signs and symptoms during hot showers. Respondents indicated that hot showers alleviated "chest congestion," "chest tightness," "chest burning," "shortness of breath," "cough," and "wheezing." Therefore, hot showers, while they may not reverse the underlying inflammation causing airway reactivity, have an effect which makes it easier for asthmatics to tolerate these reactive airways.

4. Experts in the Field Are hot showers good for asthma? Subsection 5. General Conclusions Hot showers as a treatment for asthma have never been properly investigated in clinical trials. A clinical trial was conducted in 1990 to explore the use of an inspiratory hot, humid sauna air treatment in people with severe asthma. At 10 minutes into a 30-minute treatment using hot air from an oven, some participants reported feeling better. In contrast, about 1-4 hours after the end of the treatment, 58% of the participants observed a decrease of symptoms and an increase of limitations of activities (this was bronchoconstriction).

A study conducted in 1990 on warming the airways using a hot shower suggested a possible benefit for people with asthma. However, the same study also noted that a significant proportion of people had an exacerbation of symptoms about four hours after the shower. A 2013 study "warm up and shower room effect" suggested that hot showers may have no consistent positive nor negative effects on asthma symptoms. In one group of people, cold and itchy sensation of the skin were common symptoms. Based on this evidence, we believe there may be a beneficial placebo warm-up effect, probably of short duration. This is comparable to the more pronounced reduction in asthma symptoms and increased lung function after rubbing a cream or ointment on the chest. In order to draw strong conclusions regarding the benefits of a true warm-up effect through a hot shower, we propose a comparison with a cold shower and with no shower.